A Comprehensive Guide to Effective Weight Loss

Dr. Stephanie Stiles

© 2024 by Dr. Stephanie Stiles

All Right Reserved.

Disclaimer

Each work has been made to guarantee that the data gave is exact, state-of-the-art and complete, yet no assurance is made with that impact. Moreover, the medication data contained thus might be time delicate and ought not to be used as a source of perspective asset past the date in this regard. This content does not endorse medications, diagnose patients, or suggest treatment. This information is meant to be a reference tool, not a replacement for the expertise, knowledge, and judgment of healthcare professionals who provide patient care. The shortfall of an advance notice for a given medication or blend thereof not the slightest bit ought to be understood to show wellbeing, viability, or suitability for some random patient.

Table of Contents

Introduction 1

Mild side effects 2

How does Saxenda function? 8

How should I store Saxenda? 10

How much does Saxenda cost? 12

What is the recommended dosage for Saxenda? 13

The differences between Saxenda and Victoza? 16

How to Use Saxenda 17

Precautions 21

Alcohol and Saxenda 23

How does Saxenda function? 27

What is the purpose of Saxenda? 27

Dosage Guidelines for Weight Loss in Adults: 32

Which other drugs can have an impact on Saxenda? ..35

FAQs 36

Information about Saxenda: 40

Is Saxenda similar to Ozempic? 41

Options besides Saxenda 53

Dosage for Children 56

Interactions with Saxenda 59

Taking Saxenda with meals 62

Additional precautions 66

Introduction

Saxenda is a prescription medication used for weight management. It is administered as a liquid solution in a prefilled injection pen. Saxenda is prescribed to aid in weight loss for adults and some children with obesity, as well as for overweight adults with weight-related conditions. It is intended to be part of a long-term weight management plan that includes a reduced-calorie diet and increased exercise. Saxenda contains the active ingredient liraglutide and belongs to a group of drugs known as GLP-1 agonists. Currently, Saxenda is only available as a brand-name medication and does not have a generic form.

What are the potential side effects of Saxenda?

Saxenda, like most medications, can have both mild and serious side effects. The following lists provide some examples of the more common side effects associated with Saxenda. However, it is important to note that these lists do not encompass all possible side effects that may occur when using Saxenda for weight loss.

It is important to consider that the side effects of Saxenda can vary depending on factors such as age, existing health conditions, and other medications being taken. To obtain more information about the potential side effects of Saxenda, it is recommended to consult with a doctor or pharmacist. They can also provide suggestions on how to minimize these side effects.

Mild side effects

The following is a brief list of some of the mild side effects that may be experienced when using Saxenda. To learn about other mild side effects, it is advisable to discuss with a healthcare professional or refer to Saxenda's prescribing information.

Reported mild side effects of Saxenda include:

- Vomiting

- Abdominal pain

- Upset stomach

- Constipation

- Diarrhea

- Bloating

- Fatigue (low energy)

- Dizziness

- Fever

- Injection site reactions, such as itchiness or rash in the area of injection

- Nausea

- Headache

- Mild allergic reaction

Mild side effects of many drugs may disappear within a few days to a couple of weeks. However, if they become bothersome, it is advisable to consult your doctor or pharmacist.

Although serious side effects from Saxenda can occur, they are not common. If you experience serious side effects from Saxenda, it is important to contact your doctor immediately. In the case of a medical emergency, dial 911 or your local emergency number.

Reported serious side effects of Saxenda include:

- Sudden inflammation of the pancreas (acute pancreatitis)

- Short-term gallbladder disease, such as gallstones

- Low blood sugar levels

- Faster than usual heart rate

- Kidney problems, including new or worsening kidney failure

- Suicidal thoughts or actions

- Boxed warning: Risk of thyroid cancer

- Severe allergic reaction

Focus on potential side effects of Saxenda, including a boxed warning regarding the risk of thyroid cancer. It is important to be aware of these risks and discuss them with your doctor before starting treatment. Symptoms of thyroid cancer should be monitored closely while taking Saxenda.

Before starting Saxenda, it is important to discuss your medical history with your doctor. Be sure to inform them about any existing conditions, especially those that may increase your risk of thyroid cancer, such as MTC or MEN

2. Sharing your medical history will assist your doctor in determining whether Saxenda is a safe option for you.

If you experience any symptoms of thyroid cancer while undergoing Saxenda treatment, it is crucial to contact your doctor immediately.

Nausea is a potential side effect of Saxenda. However, it is typically mild and tends to diminish as you continue using the medication.

Studies have shown that nausea is the most commonly reported side effect of Saxenda.

It is important to note that while nausea is a common side effect, it can also occur alongside more serious side effects of Saxenda, such as kidney problems, gallbladder problems, pancreatitis, and low blood sugar levels.

Tips to help with nausea caused by Saxenda include:

- Eating smaller, more frequent meals

- Avoiding rich, spicy, or greasy foods

- Drinking water regularly

- Trying ginger or peppermint teas

- Avoiding tight clothing and lying down after eating

- Staying hydrated to prevent kidney problems

If nausea is severe or persistent, it is important to consult with a doctor. Additionally, if nausea is accompanied by other symptoms like abdominal pain, fever, or decreased urination, medical attention should be sought.

Headaches may also occur during Saxenda treatment, but they are usually mild and temporary. It is important to consult with a doctor if headaches persist or worsen.

If you experience troublesome headaches while taking Saxenda, consider taking an over-the-counter pain reliever like acetaminophen (Tylenol). It is advisable to consult your doctor or pharmacist for a suitable product recommendation.

In case you have severe or persistent headaches, it is recommended to discuss the issue with your doctor.

Learn about some common questions regarding Saxenda and discover answers to them. Before starting Saxenda treatment, your doctor will assist you in creating a weight management plan that includes a low-calorie diet and increased physical activity. Working with a dietitian or nutritionist can also help tailor your plan to your specific needs.

Using Saxenda as part of your weight management plan can aid in long-term weight loss maintenance, although individual results may vary. The amount of weight lost and any potential side effects will differ from person to person.

The prescribing information for Saxenda provides information on side effects and weight loss results from clinical studies. It's important to remember that each person's experience with Saxenda will be unique.

For more information on what to expect with Saxenda, consult your doctor.

Are Wegovy, Contrave, Ozempic, Qsymia, and phentermine considered alternatives to Saxenda? Yes, most of these medications are indeed alternatives to Saxenda.

Wegovy (Semaglutide), Contrave (naltrexone/bupropion), Qsymia (phentermine/topiramate), and phentermine (Adipex-P, Lomaira) are all weight loss drugs that can be used as alternatives to Saxenda.

However, it's important to note that Ozempic (Semaglutide) is not used for weight loss. Instead, it is primarily used for the treatment of type 2 diabetes.

If you are interested in learning more about alternative options to Saxenda, it is recommended to consult with your doctor or pharmacist. Additionally, you can refer to the "Saxenda vs. Wegovy" section below for further information.

Is Saxenda available without a prescription? And does it come in pill form? No, Saxenda is not available over the counter and can only be obtained with a prescription from a healthcare professional.

Furthermore, Saxenda is not available in pill or tablet form. It is exclusively administered through injections. Oral forms of Saxenda are not available as they would not be effective due to the rapid breakdown of the drug by the digestive system.

How does Saxenda function?
Is it a form of insulin?

No, Saxenda is not classified as insulin. Insulin is a hormone that aids in the regulation of blood sugar levels. Saxenda, on the other hand, is categorized as a GLP-1 agonist medication.

GLP-1 is another hormone that assists in the management of blood sugar levels and appetite control.

Saxenda operates by mimicking the actions of GLP-1. The method by which a medication functions is referred to as its mechanism of action.

Saxenda slows down the emptying of your stomach, leading to a feeling of fullness after meals. Additionally, Saxenda helps to decrease your appetite.

By reducing calorie intake, Saxenda aids in weight management.

Can Saxenda be used to treat diabetes?

No, Saxenda is not used to treat diabetes. It is specifically used for weight loss.

Saxenda contains the same active ingredient as a diabetes medication called Victoza, which is liraglutide. However, Saxenda is prescribed at a higher dosage for weight loss compared to the dosage used for diabetes treatment with Victoza.

How should I store Saxenda?
Upon receiving a new Saxenda pen, it should be stored in the refrigerator until it is ready to be used. It is important to ensure that the pen does not freeze. Saxenda should not be used if it has been frozen.

Once you start using the new pen, you have the option to keep it at room temperature or continue storing it in the refrigerator. Regardless of the storage location, the pen remains effective for 30 days after initial use. If there is any medication left in the pen after 30 days, it should be safely disposed of.

It is important to never store the pen with a needle attached. After each dose of Saxenda, the needle should be removed and the pen cap should be replaced.

For information on how to safely dispose of needles and Saxenda pens, please refer to the manufacturer's website. If you have any further questions about Saxenda storage and disposal, it is recommended to consult with your doctor or pharmacist.

Can Saxenda be used for weight loss and weight management?

Saxenda is an injection medication used for weight loss. It is prescribed to help certain adults and children lose weight and maintain a healthy weight in the long term.

Saxenda is recommended for use in adults who have a BMI of 30 or higher (obesity) or a BMI of 27 or higher (overweight) with weight-related conditions such as high cholesterol, high blood pressure, or type 2 diabetes. It can also be used in children aged 12 and older who weigh more than 60 kilograms and have obesity based on their age, height, and sex.

This medication works by making you feel fuller after eating and reducing your appetite, leading to a decrease in calorie intake and aiding in long-term weight management. It is meant to be used as part of a comprehensive weight management plan that includes a reduced-calorie diet and increased physical activity, which your doctor can help you develop.

However, Saxenda should not be used in children with type 2 diabetes, with other weight loss products, with medications containing liraglutide or similar to Saxenda, in individuals with a history of MTC or MEN 2, in pregnant women or those who can become pregnant, or in those who have had an allergic reaction to Saxenda or its components.

How much does Saxenda cost?
The price of Saxenda can vary depending on various factors, such as your insurance coverage and the pharmacy you choose.

The monthly cost of the drug may differ for each individual, as well as the cost with or without insurance.

For more information on the cost of Saxenda, please refer to the related article.

While there is no manufacturer coupon available for Saxenda, you can explore Optum Perks coupon options in your area. By visiting Optum Perks, you can also get an estimate of the price you would pay for Saxenda when using coupons from the site.

The manufacturer of Saxenda offers resources to help you understand your insurance coverage and the treatment cost. You can visit their website to learn more.

If you have any questions regarding payment for your prescription or finding the lowest cost for Saxenda, it is recommended to consult with your doctor or pharmacist.

To discover more about saving money on prescriptions, you can also refer to this article.

What is the recommended dosage for Saxenda?
The dosage of Saxenda that is appropriate for you will be determined by your doctor. The commonly used dosages

are listed below, but it is important to always follow the dosage prescribed by your doctor.

Form and strength

Saxenda is available in the form of an injection pen. Inside the pen is a liquid solution of Saxenda that you will inject under your skin. Your doctor will provide instructions on how to administer the injection using the pen.

Saxenda strength

The Saxenda pen is available in one strength, containing 18 milligrams (mg) of liraglutide (the active drug) in 3 milliliters (mL) of solution (18 mg/3 mL). The pen can be set to inject the following doses:

0.6 mg

1.2 mg

1.8 mg

2.4 mg

3 mg

The recommended dosages for Saxenda are as follows:

- Week 1: 0.6 mg once daily

- Week 2: 1.2 mg once daily

- Week 3: 1.8 mg once daily

- Week 4: 2.4 mg once daily

- Weeks 5 and beyond: 3 mg once daily

It is important to take your dose at the same time each day. If you experience troublesome side effects after a dose increase, consult your doctor. They may suggest delaying the next dose increase for a week until the side effects improve.

The recommended maintenance dose for adults and children is 3 mg once daily. If adults experience unacceptable side effects at this dose, they may need to discontinue Saxenda treatment. Children with side effects may have their dose lowered to 2.4 mg once daily.

Common questions about Saxenda's dosage include what to do if a dose is missed, the need for long-term use, and how long it takes for Saxenda to work. If a dose is missed, it should be skipped and the next dose taken as scheduled. Extra doses should not be taken to make up for missed ones. If multiple doses are missed, a doctor should be consulted. If Saxenda is safe and effective, it may be used long term. It may take a couple of weeks to start losing weight with Saxenda, and progress should be monitored by a doctor after 4 months for adults and 3 months for children. If the recommended weight loss has not been achieved by this time, the doctor may recommend stopping treatment.

What are the differences between Saxenda and Victoza?

Both Saxenda and Victoza contain the active drug liraglutide. However, they are prescribed for different purposes. Saxenda is used for weight loss and management, while Victoza is used to treat type 2 diabetes and reduce the risk of heart issues in specific individuals.

For more information on these medications, refer to this comprehensive comparison. If you have any questions about the similarities and differences between Saxenda and Victoza, consult your doctor.

Are you curious about the differences between Saxenda and Wegovy? Saxenda contains liraglutide as its active drug, while Wegovy contains Semaglutide. Both medications are prescribed for weight loss and management.

Both Saxenda and Wegovy are administered through injections under the skin. Saxenda is taken once daily, whereas Wegovy is taken once weekly.

If you would like more details about either medication, it is advisable to consult your doctor. They will guide you in selecting the most suitable treatment option for your needs.

How to Use Saxenda

The usage of Saxenda will be explained by your doctor, including the dosage and frequency of injections. It is important to carefully follow your doctor's instructions.

Administration of Saxenda

Saxenda should be injected once daily under the skin. Your doctor will teach you how to self-administer the injection using a prefilled injection pen. Instructions can also be found on the manufacturer's website.

Injection Sites for Saxenda

You have the option to inject Saxenda into your thigh, abdomen, or upper arm. To prevent any reactions at the injection site, it is recommended to rotate the injection site with each dose. If you have any concerns or questions regarding the usage of Saxenda, consult your doctor.

Accessible Medication Containers and Labels

If you have difficulty reading the prescription label, inform your doctor or pharmacist. Some pharmacies may offer medication labels with larger print, braille, or a code that can be scanned with a smartphone to convert the text into audio. If your current pharmacy does not provide these options, your doctor or pharmacist may be able to recommend a pharmacy that does.

Combining Saxenda with other treatments

Saxenda is intended to be used as part of a comprehensive weight management strategy, which should include a reduced calorie diet and increased physical activity.

It is important to avoid using Saxenda with other weight loss products, including prescription and over-the-counter medications, herbal supplements, and weight loss products. The safety of combining Saxenda with these products is unknown.

Your doctor will not prescribe Saxenda with other medications containing liraglutide or similar drugs in the GLP-1 agonist class.

Saxenda and meal planning

Your healthcare provider can help you create a healthy, low calorie meal plan that fits your individual needs and lifestyle.

Frequently Asked Questions about Saxenda Use

Below are some common inquiries regarding the use of Saxenda:

When is the best time to inject Saxenda? You can inject Saxenda at any time of day that is most convenient for you, but it is recommended to stick to the same time daily.

Should I take Saxenda with a meal?

You can take your Saxenda dose with or without food.

Before starting Saxenda treatment, it is important to consider the following factors:

- Your overall health

- Any medical conditions you may have

- Any medications you are currently taking

- Your medical history and family medical history

It is important to discuss these considerations with your doctor before beginning Saxenda treatment. Additionally, be sure to inform your doctor about all medications, including prescription and over-the-counter drugs, as well as any vitamins, herbs, or supplements you are taking. This will help to identify any potential interactions that may affect how Saxenda works.

Do not use Saxenda with certain drugs, herbs, or supplements. These include other GLP-1 agonists like Saxenda (dulaglutide, other forms of liraglutide, Semaglutide), as well as other weight loss products (Orlistat, phentermine, phentermine / topiramate, naltrexone / bupropion, chitosan, chromium, ephedra, Garcinia camogie, green tea, guar gum, mangos teen, modified cellulose, pyruvate). Saxenda can also interact with insulin, sulfonylurea drugs for diabetes, and medications taken orally. This is not an exhaustive list, so consult your doctor or pharmacist for more information on potential interactions with Saxenda.

Boxed Warning: Saxenda carries a serious warning from the FDA regarding potential dangerous effects of the drug.

Thyroid Cancer Risk: Saxenda may pose a potential risk of thyroid cancer. Animal studies have shown that the active ingredient, liraglutide, can cause thyroid tumors. However, it is uncertain whether the drug has the same effect on humans.

Precautions: Your doctor is unlikely to prescribe Saxenda if you or a close family member has a rare form of thyroid cancer known as medullary thyroid cancer, or if you have a rare inherited condition called multiple endocrine neoplasia syndrome type 2 (MEN 2), which increases your risk of thyroid cancer.

Precautions

Before starting Saxenda treatment, it is important to discuss your medical history with your doctor to determine if it is the right option for you.

Factors to consider include the following:

- Allergic reactions: If you have had an allergic reaction to Saxenda or any of its ingredients, your doctor may not prescribe it. Ask about alternative medications.

- Kidney problems: Saxenda could worsen kidney problems such as kidney failure. Consult with your doctor to see if it is safe for you.

- Liver problems: Saxenda has not been extensively studied in individuals with liver issues. Discuss with your doctor if it is safe for you.

- History of pancreatitis: In rare cases, Saxenda may cause acute pancreatitis. Inform your doctor if you have a history of pancreatitis to determine if Saxenda is suitable for you.

- Slow stomach emptying: Saxenda can slow down stomach emptying. If you have this condition, talk to your doctor about its safety for you.

- Type 2 diabetes: Saxenda may cause low blood sugar levels, especially in adults with type 2 diabetes who take certain medications. Your doctor may need to adjust your diabetes medication before starting Saxenda.

- Depression or suicidal thoughts: In rare cases, Saxenda may lead to suicidal thoughts. If you have a history of depression or suicidal tendencies, your doctor may not prescribe Saxenda. Discuss your mental health history with your doctor before starting treatment.

Alcohol and Saxenda

Consuming alcohol while taking Saxenda may exacerbate certain side effects such as headaches, nausea, vomiting, diarrhea, upset stomach, dizziness, and low blood sugar levels. Additionally, excessive alcohol intake can lead to dehydration, increasing the risk of kidney issues when using Saxenda.

If you drink alcohol, it is important to consult your doctor to determine if it is safe to do so while on Saxenda.

Pregnancy and Nursing

Saxenda should not be used during pregnancy as weight loss during this time can be harmful to the developing fetus. If you become pregnant while on Saxenda, discontinue use and contact your doctor immediately.

If you are planning to become pregnant, discuss safe weight management options with your doctor.

It is unclear whether Saxenda passes into breast milk. If you are breastfeeding or planning to breastfeed, speak with your doctor about the potential benefits and risks of using Saxenda.

In the event of an overdose, it is important to avoid injecting more Saxenda than prescribed by your doctor. Injecting an excessive amount can result in severe side effects.

Signs of an overdose may include:

- Intense nausea

- Severe vomiting

- Significantly low blood sugar levels, leading to:

  - Dizziness

  - Tremors

  - Blurred vision

  - Rapid heartbeat

  - Excessive sweating

  - Irritability

  - Confusion

  - Weakness

  - Impaired coordination

- Difficulty swallowing

- Loss of consciousness

If you have any questions about Saxenda treatment, it is recommended to consult with your doctor. They can provide information on various weight management options and help determine if Saxenda is suitable for you.

Some questions you may want to ask your doctor regarding Saxenda treatment are:

- What should I do if I am not experiencing weight loss with Saxenda?

- Will I need to continue using Saxenda even after reaching my target weight?

- Are there any potential long-term side effects associated with Saxenda?

For additional resources on weight management, the following articles may be helpful:

- "Ask the Expert: 9 Things to Consider in a Weight Management Program for Obesity"

- "Treatments to Manage Obesity: What Works and What Doesn't?"

To stay informed about different health conditions and receive tips for improving your well-being, consider subscribing to Health line's newsletters. Additionally, you may find support and connect with others in the online communities at Buzzy, a platform designed for individuals with specific health conditions.

Saxenda (liraglutide) is a medication used to aid in weight loss and weight maintenance in obese or overweight adults with weight-related medical issues. It can also be used in adolescents aged 12 to 17 years who are obese and have a bodyweight above 132 pounds (60 kg). Saxenda is meant to be used alongside a healthy diet and exercise regimen.

This medication is administered through a once-daily injection under the skin using a multi-dose injection pen.

Saxenda contains the same active ingredient (liraglutide) as Victoza. However, Saxenda and Victoza differ in their strengths and are approved by the FDA for different conditions.

It is important to note that Saxenda is not intended for the treatment of type 1 or type 2 diabetes. Its safety and effectiveness have not been established in children under 12 years of age or in adolescents aged 12 to 17 years with type 2 diabetes.

How does Saxenda function?
Saxenda operates by reducing appetite, slowing down gastric emptying, and prolonging the feeling of fullness, resulting in a decrease in calorie intake. It mimics a hormone naturally found in the body that helps regulate blood sugar, insulin levels, and digestion. Saxenda falls under the category of medications known as glucagon-like peptide-1 (GLP-1) agonists.

What is the purpose of Saxenda?
Saxenda has been approved by the FDA for weight loss and for maintaining weight loss after initial success. It can be used in the following cases:

For adults:

- Obese adults with a BMI of 30 kg/m2 or higher.

- Overweight adults with a BMI of 27 kg/m2 or higher, who also have weight-related medical conditions such as hypertension, type 2 diabetes mellitus, or dyslipidemia.

For pediatric patients aged 12 years and older:

- Those with a body weight exceeding 60 kg.

- Those with an initial BMI corresponding to 30 kg/m2 or higher for adults (classified as obese according to international cut-offs, specifically the Cole Criteria).

Before starting Saxenda, it is important to consider certain factors. Saxenda should not be used if you are allergic to liraglutide or if you have multiple endocrine neoplasia type 2, a personal or family history of medullary thyroid carcinoma, or diabetic ketoacidosis. Additionally, if you are using insulin or other medications like liraglutide, Saxenda should not be used. To ensure the safety of Saxenda, inform your doctor if you have stomach problems causing slow digestion, kidney or liver disease, high triglycerides, heart problems, a history of pancreas or gallbladder issues, or a history of depression or suicidal thoughts. Animal studies have shown that liraglutide may cause thyroid tumors or thyroid cancer, but it is unclear if this would occur in humans using regular doses. If you are pregnant or planning to become pregnant, it is unknown if Saxenda could harm an unborn baby, so it is important to inform your doctor. Similarly, it is unclear if liraglutide passes into breast milk or affects nursing babies, so inform your doctor if you are breastfeeding. Lastly, Saxenda is not approved for use in individuals under 18 years old according to the FDA.

How to properly use Saxenda:

Saxenda is typically administered once a day. It is important to follow the instructions on your prescription label and your doctor may adjust your dose as needed. Do not exceed the recommended dosage or use the medication for a longer period than prescribed.

It is not recommended to use Saxenda and Victoza together, as they contain the same active ingredient.

Make sure to read all provided patient information, medication guides, and instruction sheets. If you have any questions, consult your doctor or pharmacist.

Saxenda should be injected under the skin at any time of the day, with or without a meal. You will be taught how to administer the injections at home. Do not self-inject if you are unsure of the proper technique or how to dispose of used needles and syringes.

The medication comes in a prefilled injection pen. Ask your pharmacist for advice on which needles are best suited for use with your pen.

Your healthcare provider will advise you on the best injection sites on your body. Rotate the injection site each time and avoid injecting in the same spot consecutively.

Do not use Saxenda if it has changed color or contains particles. Contact your pharmacist for a replacement.

Be aware of symptoms of high blood sugar, such as increased thirst or urination, blurred vision, headache, and fatigue.

Various factors can affect blood sugar levels, including stress, illness, surgery, exercise, alcohol consumption, or skipping meals. Consult your doctor before making any changes to your dosage or medication schedule.

Use a disposable needle only once and dispose of it according to state and local laws. Use a puncture-proof "sharps" disposal container, which can be obtained from your pharmacist. Keep the container out of reach of children and pets.

Saxenda is just one part of a comprehensive treatment plan that may include diet, exercise, weight management, regular blood sugar monitoring, and specialized medical care. It is important to follow your doctor's instructions carefully.

When storing unopened injection pens, keep them in the refrigerator and do not freeze them. Discard any medication that has been frozen or has passed the expiration date. After the first use, "in-use" injection pens can be stored in the refrigerator or at room temperature for up to 30 days.

Protect them from moisture, heat, and sunlight, and remember to remove the needle before storing. Keep the cap on the pen when not in use.

Dosage Guidelines for Weight Loss in Adults:

To minimize gastrointestinal symptoms, it is recommended to gradually increase the dose. If needed, the dose escalation can be delayed by one week:

- Week 1: Administer 0.6 mg subcutaneously once daily

- Week 2: Administer 1.2 mg subcutaneously once daily

- Week 3: Administer 1.8 mg subcutaneously once daily

- Week 4: Administer 2.4 mg subcutaneously once daily

- Week 5: Administer 3 mg subcutaneously once daily

Maintenance Dose:

Administer 3 mg subcutaneously once daily. If the maintenance dose is not well-tolerated, it is recommended to discontinue use. The effectiveness of chronic weight management at lower doses has not been established.

Additional Information:

Do not use Saxenda in combination with any other GLP-1 receptor agonist. The safety and efficacy of Saxenda in combination with other weight loss products, including prescription drugs, over-the-counter drugs, and herbal supplements, have not been determined.

Evaluate weight loss progress at 16 weeks. If the patient has not lost at least 4% of their body weight, it is unlikely that they will achieve significant and sustained weight loss with continued treatment.

Indication: Saxenda is used as an adjunct to a reduced-calorie diet and increased physical activity for chronic weight management in adult patients with an initial BMI of 30 kg/m2 or higher (obese) or an initial BMI of 27 kg/m2 or higher (overweight) with at least one weight-related comorbid condition (e.g., hypertension, type 2 diabetes mellitus, or dyslipidemia).

BMI (Body Mass Index) is calculated by dividing weight in kilograms by height in meters squared. Charts are available to determine BMI based on height and weight, including a chart in the Saxenda product labeling.

Typical Pediatric Dosage for Weight Loss:

For children aged 12 and older:

To minimize the chances of experiencing gastrointestinal symptoms, it is recommended to gradually increase the dosage. If necessary, the dosage escalation can be delayed based on tolerability. The process of increasing the dosage may take up to 8 weeks:

Week 1: Administer 0.6 mg subcutaneously once daily

Week 2: Administer 1.2 mg subcutaneously once daily

Week 3: Administer 1.8 mg subcutaneously once daily

Week 4: Administer 2.4 mg subcutaneously once daily

Week 5: Administer 3 mg subcutaneously once daily

What occurs if I forget to take a dose?

If you forget to take your daily dose of Saxenda, take it as soon as you remember. Then continue with your regular daily dose the next day. Do not take an additional dose of Saxenda or increase your dose the next day to compensate for the missed dose.

If you forget to take your dose of Saxenda for three days or more, contact your healthcare provider to discuss how to resume your treatment.

To ensure safe use of Saxenda, avoid sharing injection pens, cartridges, or syringes with others to prevent the spread of infections or diseases. Additionally, do not combine Saxenda with other weight loss products, diet pills, or appetite suppressants.

If you experience signs of an allergic reaction to Saxenda such as hives, fast heartbeats, dizziness, trouble breathing or swallowing, or swelling of the face, lips, tongue, or throat, seek immediate medical attention. Contact your doctor right away if you notice any concerning symptoms, including racing or pounding heartbeats, sudden changes in mood or behavior, severe nausea, vomiting, diarrhea, or any other serious side effects listed above.

Which other drugs can have an impact on Saxenda?

Saxenda has the potential to slow down digestion and may result in a longer absorption time for orally taken medications.

Inform your doctor about all the medications you are currently taking, as well as any new ones you start or stop using. Pay particular attention to:

- Insulin

- Oral diabetes medications such as Glucotrol, Metaglip, Amaryl, Avandaryl, Duetact, DiaBeta, Micronase, Glucovance, and others.

Please note that this list is not exhaustive. Liraglutide, the active ingredient in Saxenda, may interact with other prescription and over-the-counter drugs, as well as vitamins and herbal products. This medication guide does not include all possible interactions.

FAQs
How does Saxenda function?

Saxenda operates by controlling hunger and calorie intake for weight loss. As a glucagon-like peptide 1 (GLP-1) receptor agonist, it reduces hunger signals in various parts of the brain, leading to a decrease in food consumption.

Saxenda also slows down the digestion of food in the stomach, creating a sensation of fullness. However, this can interact with certain medications, so it is essential to discuss all your medications with your healthcare provider.

Additionally, it boosts insulin secretion, aiding in the absorption of glucose by cells for energy. It also reduces glucagon secretion in the body, which helps in lowering blood glucose levels.

Does Saxenda require refrigeration?

Unopened Saxenda pens should be stored in the refrigerator at temperatures between 36°F to 46°F. Do not freeze. After the initial injection, Saxenda can be refrigerated or kept at room temperature (59°F to 86°F) for up to 30 days. Ensure the pen is not exposed to direct heat or sunlight.

How long is a Saxenda pen effective?

A Saxenda pen can be used for 30 days. After this period, the medication expires and should be discarded, even if there is still medicine left. The duration of each pen depends on the dosage taken, with a scale on the pen indicating the remaining Saxenda.

What is the typical weight loss with Saxenda?

In clinical trials, a higher percentage of individuals who used Saxenda for 56 weeks lost 5 to 10% of their body weight compared to those on a placebo. This equates to a weight loss of 12 to 23 pounds. Participants in the studies were either overweight or obese before starting Saxenda.

Can Saxenda be consumed with alcohol?

There are no specific warnings about consuming alcohol while taking Saxenda. However, alcohol can lower blood sugar levels, increasing the risk of hypoglycemia when combined with other diabetes medications. Alcoholic beverages are also high in carbohydrates and sugar, which may hinder weight loss efforts.

How long does it take for Saxenda to take effect?

Saxenda reaches peak concentration in the body 11 hours after injection. It is advisable to follow up with your doctor 2 to 8 weeks after starting Saxenda to assess its effectiveness.

If you have not lost 4% of your body weight after 16 weeks, your doctor may recommend discontinuing the medication. In children aged 12 and above, Saxenda may be stopped after 12 weeks on the maintenance dose if BMI has not decreased by 1%.

Saxenda is a subcutaneous injection that is prescribed under the brand name for weight management in certain individuals. It contains liraglutide, an active drug, and falls under the drug class of glucagon-like peptide-1 (GLP-1) agonists.

Saxenda has been approved by the FDA to aid in weight loss and long-term weight management when used in conjunction with a reduced-calorie diet and increased exercise. Specifically, it is approved for use in the following groups:

- Adults who meet either of the following criteria:

 - Individuals with obesity, defined as a body mass index (BMI) of 30 or higher.

 - Individuals who are overweight (with a BMI of 27 or higher) and have a weight-related condition such as type 2 diabetes, high blood pressure, or high cholesterol.

- Children aged 12 years and older who meet the following criteria:

 - Weigh more than 60 kilograms (approximately 132 pounds).

 - Have obesity based on their age, sex, and height, equivalent to an adult BMI of 30 or higher.

Information about Saxenda:
- Drug class: GLP-1 agonist

- Form: liquid solution for subcutaneous injection with prefilled pen

- Generic available: No

- Prescription required: Yes

- Controlled substance: No

- FDA approval year: 2010

There is currently no generic version of Saxenda available. Saxenda is only sold as a brand-name medication. Generic drugs are identical copies of the active drug in a brand-name medication and are typically cheaper than brand-name drugs.

The cost of Saxenda can vary, depending on factors such as your insurance plan, location, and pharmacy. You can visit Optum Perks for price estimates using their coupons, but please note that these coupons cannot be used with insurance copays or benefits. If you need financial assistance or help understanding your insurance coverage for Saxenda, the manufacturer offers support on their website. Saxenda does not have a generic version available, as generics are typically cheaper alternatives to brand-name drugs.

Are there any reviews from individuals who have used Saxenda? Where can I locate before and after photos?

Online reviews from Saxenda users may be accessible. However, it is important to note that each person's experience with Saxenda will vary. The amount of weight one may lose and any potential side effects are dependent on individual circumstances.

Is Saxenda similar to Ozempic?

Yes, Saxenda and Ozempic are both part of the same drug class known as glucagon-like peptide-1 (GLP-1) agonists. GLP-1 agonists work by increasing insulin levels and reducing appetite. However, they have different approved uses. Saxenda is used for weight management, while Ozempic is used to treat type 2 diabetes and reduce the risk of cardiovascular problems in certain adults. Saxenda contains liraglutide as its active drug, while Ozempic contains Semaglutide. Another brand-name version of Semaglutide called Wegovy is also available for weight loss and management. Both Saxenda and Wegovy are administered through injections, but Saxenda is taken once daily while Wegovy is taken once weekly. For more information on how Saxenda compares to similar drugs, consult your doctor or pharmacist.

Is Saxenda available in pill form, like tablets?

No, Saxenda is not available in pill form. It is only offered as a liquid solution in an injection pen.

Saxenda contains liraglutide, a protein-based drug. If taken orally, it would be rapidly broken down by the digestive system, rendering it ineffective.

Researchers are exploring alternative forms of protein-based drugs that can be taken orally. However, at present, Saxenda must be administered via injection.

Is Saxenda a form of insulin?

No, Saxenda is not a form of insulin. It belongs to a drug class known as GLP-1 agonists and contains the active drug liraglutide.

Insulin is a hormone produced by the body to regulate blood sugar levels. People with diabetes either do not produce enough insulin or do not use it effectively. Synthetic forms of insulin are used to help manage blood sugar levels in individuals with diabetes.

GLP-1 agonists, like insulin, are used to treat diabetes. They stimulate the production of insulin in the body but are not classified as insulin. Liraglutide (Victoza) is an example of a GLP-1 agonist approved for diabetes treatment. While Saxenda is not approved for diabetes treatment, it may assist in increasing insulin production in the body.

If you are not seeing weight loss results with Saxenda, it is important to speak with your doctor. While immediate results should not be expected, if you are not losing weight within the first 4 months of treatment, your doctor can assess if you are using the medication correctly or if there are issues with your diet and exercise plan.

Your doctor will schedule an appointment 4 months after starting treatment to monitor your progress. By this point, adults should ideally have lost at least 4% of their body weight, while children should have a lower BMI by at least 1%.

If you or your child have not achieved the expected weight loss after the specified time frame, it may indicate that

Saxenda is not effective for you. In such cases, your doctor may recommend exploring alternative treatment options.

Saxenda is an FDA-approved prescription drug that is used to treat certain conditions. It is specifically approved for weight loss and long-term weight management in individuals who are obese or overweight and have certain weight-related conditions. Saxenda is used in conjunction with a reduced-calorie diet and increased exercise. It is approved for use in adults who have a body mass index (BMI) of 30 or more, or a BMI of 27 or more with a weight-related condition such as type 2 diabetes, high blood pressure, or high cholesterol. It is also approved for use in children aged 12 and older who weigh more than 60 kilograms and have obesity based on their age, sex, and height. Saxenda works by reducing appetite and is meant to be used as part of a long-term weight management plan. Your doctor can help you develop a plan that suits your needs and can provide guidance on healthy ways to reduce calorie intake and increase physical activity.

Restrictions on use

Saxenda should not be combined with other glucagon-like peptide-1 (GLP-1) agonists, as they belong to the same drug group.

The safety and effectiveness of Saxenda in children with type 2 diabetes is unknown.

Furthermore, Saxenda was not tested in individuals using weight loss products like other prescription drugs, over-the-counter drugs, or herbal supplements. Therefore, it is unclear if Saxenda is safe or effective when used in conjunction with these products.

Saxenda is a proven medication for achieving weight loss and managing weight in individuals with obesity and some who are overweight. It is recommended in the guidelines for obesity management by the American Diabetes Association and the American Association of Clinical Endocrinologists. For more information on the drug's effectiveness in clinical trials, refer to Saxenda's prescribing information.

Saxenda is approved by the FDA for weight loss and long-term weight management in children aged 12 and above who weigh over 60 kg (approximately 132 pounds) and have obesity based on their age, sex, and height (equivalent to an adult BMI of 30 or higher). It is not recommended for children under 12 years old or those with type 2 diabetes. The safety and effectiveness of Saxenda in these groups of children is unknown.

It is recommended to incorporate Saxenda into a comprehensive weight management strategy that involves a low-calorie diet and regular physical activity. Avoid combining Saxenda with other weight loss medications, over-the-counter drugs, or herbal supplements, as the safety and effectiveness of such combinations are unknown.

If you are considering Saxenda, it is advisable to consult with your doctor, dietitian, or nutritionist to create a personalized meal or diet plan. They can assist you in finding the most suitable approach for your needs. Additionally, discussing with your doctor about effective methods to decrease calorie consumption and enhance physical activity can be beneficial for your overall health.

There are potential mild or severe side effects associated with Saxenda. The following lists outline some of the main side effects that may occur when using Saxenda. Please note that these lists are not exhaustive and other side effects may also occur.

To learn more about potential side effects of Saxenda, consult your healthcare provider or pharmacist. They can provide guidance on how to address any bothersome side effects. Additionally, you can refer to this article for further information on Saxenda's side effects. Please note that the FDA monitors drug side effects and you can report any issues you experience with Saxenda to the FDA through Med Watch.

Common side effects of Saxenda may include:

- Nausea

- Vomiting

- Diarrhea

- Constipation

- Indigestion

- Abdominal pain

- Bloating

- Gas

- Injection site reactions

- Headache

- Fatigue

- Dizziness

- Gastroenteritis

These side effects are usually mild and may resolve within a few days to a couple of weeks. If they persist or worsen, it is recommended to consult with a healthcare professional.

Severe side effects

Although rare, serious side effects can occur while taking Saxenda. If you experience any of these symptoms, contact your doctor immediately. In case of life-threatening symptoms or a medical emergency, call 911 or your local emergency services.

Serious side effects may include:

- Hypoglycemia (low blood sugar): symptoms may include dizziness, shakiness, blurred vision, nausea, irritability, confusion, hunger, fast heart rate, and sweating.

- Increased heart rate: symptoms may include racing or pounding sensations in the heart.

- Acute pancreatitis: symptoms may include severe abdominal pain, nausea, vomiting, and fever.

- Gallbladder problems: symptoms may include abdominal pain, nausea, vomiting, fever, diarrhea, pale stools, and jaundice.

- Kidney failure: symptoms may include decreased urination, swelling of ankles and feet, nausea, confusion, and shortness of breath.

- Suicidal thoughts or actions: symptoms may include new or worsening depression, thoughts of self-harm, or changes in mood or behavior.

- Allergic reaction.

- Risk of thyroid cancer.

Side effects in children using Saxenda are comparable to those experienced by adults. Some children may also experience a fever while taking this medication. In clinical trials, children were more likely to experience hypoglycemia and gastroenteritis compared to adults. If you have any concerns about the potential side effects of Saxenda in children, consult with your child's doctor for more information.

Detailed information on potential side effects

This medication, Saxenda, contains liraglutide which has been shown to cause certain types of thyroid cancer in animal studies. However, it is unclear whether Saxenda poses a risk of thyroid cancer in humans.

Due to the potential risk of thyroid cancer associated with Saxenda, the medication carries a boxed warning about this side effect. A boxed warning is the most severe warning issued by the FDA, alerting healthcare providers and patients about potentially dangerous effects of the drug.

Your healthcare provider will not prescribe Saxenda if you or a close family member has a history of a rare form of thyroid cancer known as medullary thyroid cancer. Close family members include parents, siblings, or children. Additionally, Saxenda will not be prescribed if you have a rare genetic condition called multiple endocrine neoplasia syndrome type 2 (MEN 2), which increases the risk of thyroid cancer.

If you experience symptoms of thyroid cancer while taking Saxenda, it is important to contact your doctor immediately. These symptoms may include a lump in your neck, a persistent hoarse voice, difficulty swallowing, or shortness of breath. If you are diagnosed with thyroid cancer, your doctor will advise you to discontinue the use of Saxenda.

Some individuals may experience side effects at the injection site when using Saxenda. These are known as injection site reactions and were commonly observed in clinical trials. Typically, these reactions are mild and may include changes in skin color, such as redness, darkening, or discoloration, swelling, itching, skin rash, or pain.

To minimize the occurrence of injection site reactions, it is recommended to inject Saxenda at least one finger width away from the previous injection spot or choose a different area of the body for each injection. Suitable injection sites include the abdomen, thigh, and upper arm. After administering Saxenda, avoid rubbing the injection site.

If you do experience an injection site reaction, it should improve within a few days. Refrain from injecting Saxenda in that particular area until the reaction subsides. If the reaction is bothersome, applying a cold pack to the area may provide relief. However, if the reaction is severe or does not improve, it is advisable to consult your doctor.

Nausea is a common side effect of taking Saxenda, as it can slow down the passage of food through your stomach and cause bloating. However, this side effect is usually mild and tends to improve as your body adjusts to the medication.

If you experience nausea while taking Saxenda, you can try eating bland foods, avoiding lying down after eating, staying hydrated, drinking ginger or peppermint tea, getting fresh air, and avoiding tight clothing. It's important to drink plenty of fluids to prevent dehydration, which can increase the risk of kidney problems.

While nausea is a common side effect, it can also be a symptom of more serious issues such as gallbladder problems, pancreatitis, or kidney problems. If your nausea is severe or persistent, it's important to speak with your doctor to rule out any serious side effects and explore other ways to manage this symptom.

Saxenda and Victoza share the same active ingredient, liraglutide, but they are prescribed for different purposes. Saxenda is prescribed for weight loss, whereas Victoza is prescribed for type 2 diabetes and to reduce the likelihood of severe cardiovascular issues in specific adults.

Options besides Saxenda

There are various medications available for weight loss and weight management that may suit you better. If you are considering an alternative to Saxenda, consult with your doctor. They can provide information on other drugs that could be effective for you.

Some examples of alternative medications for weight loss and weight management are:

- Orlistat (Alli, Xenical)

- Phentermine (Adipex-P, Lomaira)

- Phentermine/topiramate (Qsymia)

- Naltrexone/bupropion (Contrave)

- Semaglutide (Wegovy)

The dosage of Saxenda will be gradually increased by your doctor when you begin treatment. This is done to help your body adjust to the medication and minimize the chances of experiencing digestive system side effects. It is important to follow the dosage prescribed by your doctor, as they will determine the most suitable dosage for you.

Saxenda is available in the form of a liquid solution, administered through subcutaneous injection. It is conveniently packaged in a prefilled injection pen. Each pen contains 18 milligrams of liraglutide in a 3 milliliter solution (18 mg/3 mL). The pen allows for adjustable dosing options, with settings for 0.6 mg, 1.2 mg, 1.8 mg, 2.4 mg, and 3 mg.

Dosage for weight loss and weight management

To begin treatment with Saxenda for weight loss, it is typically recommended to start with a dosage of 0.6 mg once daily for the first week. The dosage is then increased gradually for each subsequent week:

- Week two: 1.2 mg daily

- Week three: 1.8 mg daily

- Week four: 2.4 mg daily

- Week five and beyond: 3 mg daily

If you experience troublesome side effects after an increase in dosage, it is important to consult with your doctor. They may suggest delaying the next scheduled dosage increase for about a week to allow the side effects to diminish.

For long-term weight management in adults, the recommended maintenance dosage is 3 mg daily. If you are unable to tolerate the side effects at this dosage, your doctor may advise discontinuing Saxenda treatment.

Dosage for Children

For children aged 12 years and older starting treatment with Saxenda, it is recommended to begin with the same dosage as adults. Their dosage should be gradually increased as outlined earlier.

If a child experiences troublesome side effects following an increase in dosage, it is advisable to consult their doctor. The doctor may suggest postponing the next planned dosage increase for approximately one week to allow the side effects to diminish. It can take up to 8 weeks for children to reach the recommended maintenance dosage.

Just like adults, children are typically recommended to take a maintenance dosage of 3 mg per day. However, if a child experiences side effects that are too severe at this dosage, a lower maintenance dosage of 2.4 mg per day may be prescribed. If the child still cannot tolerate the side effects at this lower dosage, their doctor will likely advise discontinuing their Saxenda treatment.

What should I do if I forget to take a dose?

If you forget to take a dose of Saxenda, simply skip the missed dose and stick to your regular dosing schedule. It is important not to take an additional dose to compensate for the missed one, as this can increase the likelihood of experiencing side effects from the medication.

If you fail to take Saxenda for more than three doses, it is advisable to consult your doctor. They will probably recommend restarting your Saxenda treatment with a daily dose of 0.6 mg for one week. Your doctor will then gradually increase the dosage each week, as previously done, until you reach your regular maintenance dosage.

To avoid missing a dose, consider using a medication reminder. This can involve setting an alarm or timer, or downloading a reminder app on your phone.

There is no known interaction between Saxenda and alcohol. However, consuming alcohol while taking Saxenda may worsen certain side effects such as nausea, diarrhea, dizziness, headache, fatigue, and hypoglycemia. Additionally, alcohol can lead to dehydration, increasing the risk of kidney problems when taking Saxenda. It is important to discuss with your doctor how much, if any, alcohol is safe to consume while on Saxenda.

It is not recommended to use Saxenda during pregnancy as its effects on human pregnancy have not been studied. Saxenda is typically used for weight loss and management in specific individuals, but losing weight while pregnant can potentially harm the fetus.

In animal trials, Saxenda administration to pregnant females resulted in the development of birth defects. However, it is important to note that the outcomes of animal trials may not always reflect what will occur in humans.

If you discover that you are pregnant while taking Saxenda, it is advised to discontinue its use and consult your doctor.

If you are sexually active and there is a possibility of pregnancy, it is important to discuss your birth control options with your doctor while using Saxenda, as it is not recommended for use during pregnancy.

The safety of using Saxenda while breastfeeding is uncertain as it is unclear if the drug can pass into breast milk or have any impact on a nursing baby. If you are currently breastfeeding or intend to breastfeed, it is advisable to consult your doctor to determine if Saxenda is suitable for you.

Interactions with Saxenda

There are various medications that can interact with Saxenda. These interactions may have different effects. For example, some interactions can impact the effectiveness of a medication, while others can amplify side effects or make them more intense.

Saxenda and other medications

The following is a partial list of medications that may interact with Saxenda. It is not exhaustive.

Prior to taking Saxenda, it is important to consult with your doctor and pharmacist. Inform them of all prescription, over-the-counter (OTC), and other medications you are currently taking. Additionally, disclose any vitamins, herbs, or supplements you are using. Providing this information can help prevent potential interactions.

If you have any concerns about how drug interactions may impact you, do not hesitate to ask your doctor or pharmacist.

Do not take Saxenda with other GLP-1 agonists such as dulaglutide, Victoza, or Semaglutide. It is also not recommended to use Saxenda with other weight loss drugs like Orlistat, phentermine, phentermine/topiramate, or naltrexone/bupropion.

Other drugs that may interact with Saxenda include certain diabetes medications. Taking Saxenda with insulin or sulfonylureas can increase the risk of low blood sugar. Examples of these medications include Novolog, Humalog, Levemir, Toujeo, Humulin R, Novolin R, Humulin N, Novolin N, Glucotrol, Amaryl, Diabeta, and Glynase. Additionally, medications taken orally, such as tablets, capsules, pills, or liquids, may take longer to be absorbed when taken with Saxenda. It is important to consult with your doctor or pharmacist if you take any oral medications to determine if they may be affected by Saxenda.

It is not recommended to use Saxenda in combination with herbal weight loss products or supplements, as the safety of this combination is unknown. Examples of such products include green tea, ephedra, guar gum, chitosan, chromium, Garcinia cambogia, mangosteen, modified cellulose, and pyruvate. While there are no other reported interactions between Saxenda and herbs or supplements, it is still advisable to consult with your doctor or pharmacist before using any of these products while taking Saxenda.

To properly use Saxenda, follow the instructions provided by your doctor. Saxenda is administered through subcutaneous injection, which means it is injected just under the skin. Your doctor will guide you on how to use the Saxenda pen for self-injection at home. Additionally, the manufacturer's website offers comprehensive instructions and a step-by-step video.

Injection sites for Saxenda include the abdomen, thigh, or upper arm. It is important to rotate these sites with each dose. For instance, if you inject Saxenda into one area of your abdomen, the next dose should be administered in a different area of the abdomen (at least one finger width away), or in the thigh or upper arm.

When to administer Saxenda

It is recommended to inject Saxenda once daily at a time that is convenient for you. It is best to use Saxenda at the same time each day to maintain consistency.

To avoid missing a dose, consider using a medication reminder such as setting an alarm or timer. You may also find it helpful to download a reminder app on your phone.

Taking Saxenda with meals

You have the option to take your Saxenda injection with or without food.

Saxenda functions by aiding in weight loss and maintaining a healthy weight over the long term for individuals with obesity and some overweight individuals. This medication is taken alongside a reduced-calorie diet and increased physical activity.

The occurrence of overweight and obesity is typically a result of consuming more calories than one burns. This can lead to weight gain over time.

To combat this, adopting a reduced-calorie diet and increasing physical activity can aid in weight loss. However, in some cases, making these lifestyle changes may not be sufficient for long-term weight loss maintenance. One reason for this is that a reduced-calorie diet can increase feelings of hunger and reduce feelings of fullness. Consequently, individuals may continue to consume more calories than they can burn through physical activity, hindering weight loss progress.

Saxenda aids in weight loss by reducing appetite and promoting a feeling of fullness after meals. Its active ingredient, liraglutide, is classified as a glucagon-like peptide-1 (GLP-1) agonist.

GLP-1 is a hormone that regulates appetite and blood sugar levels. By binding to GLP-1 receptors in the brain, it produces various effects. These include decreased hunger and slowed digestion, leading to a greater sense of satiety after eating.

Saxenda mimics the structure of GLP-1, functioning similarly to the natural hormone in the body. By helping to reduce calorie intake, Saxenda supports long-term weight loss maintenance.

How long does it take for Saxenda to take effect? Saxenda typically starts working a few hours after the first dose is injected, but it may take one to two weeks before weight loss begins.

Your doctor will evaluate your progress four months after starting treatment to determine if Saxenda is effective for you. Typically, adults should have lost at least 4% of their body weight by this time.

For children, a doctor's appointment will be scheduled three months after starting treatment. At this point, children are expected to have a body mass index (BMI) that is at least 1% lower than when they began treatment.

If you or your child have not achieved the expected amount of weight loss within the appropriate timeframe, it is unlikely that Saxenda is effective for you.

FDA warning: Increased risk of thyroid cancer

This medication carries a boxed warning, which is the most severe warning issued by the Food and Drug Administration (FDA). A boxed warning is intended to inform doctors and patients about potentially dangerous side effects of the drug.

The active ingredient in Saxenda, known as Liraglutide, has been found to cause certain types of thyroid cancer in animals. However, it is currently unknown whether Saxenda increases the risk of thyroid cancer in humans.

Due to this risk, your doctor will not prescribe Saxenda if you or a close family member has a history of medullary thyroid cancer. Additionally, Saxenda will not be prescribed if you have a rare genetic condition called multiple endocrine neoplasia syndrome type 2 (MEN 2), as this condition heightens the risk of thyroid cancer.

If you experience any symptoms of thyroid cancer while taking Saxenda, such as a lump in your neck, persistent hoarseness, difficulty swallowing, or shortness of breath, it is important to notify your doctor immediately.

Additional precautions

Prior to starting Saxenda, it is important to discuss your medical history with your doctor. Saxenda may not be suitable for individuals with certain medical conditions or factors that may impact their health.

These conditions and factors include:

- Allergic reaction: If you have previously experienced an allergic reaction to Saxenda or any of its ingredients, your doctor will not prescribe this medication. It is recommended to consult your doctor about alternative medications that may be more suitable for you.

- Type 2 diabetes: Saxenda can potentially cause hypoglycemia. Individuals with type 2 diabetes who take insulin or sulfonylureas are at a higher risk of experiencing this side effect. If you have type 2 diabetes, it is important to discuss this with your doctor. They may monitor your blood sugar levels before starting Saxenda and adjust your diabetes medication dosage accordingly. Regular blood sugar monitoring may also be necessary while taking Saxenda. It is important to note that Saxenda should not be used in children with type 2 diabetes, as its safety and effectiveness in this population are unknown.

- Pancreatitis: In rare cases, Saxenda may lead to pancreatitis, which is inflammation of the pancreas. If you have a history of pancreatitis or currently have this condition, it is uncertain whether you have an increased risk of experiencing this side effect with Saxenda. It is advisable to consult your doctor to determine if Saxenda is appropriate for you.

- Kidney problems: Saxenda may rarely cause or worsen kidney failure. If you have kidney problems, it is important to discuss with your doctor whether Saxenda is suitable for you. Additionally, it is recommended to stay well-hydrated while taking Saxenda, especially if you experience vomiting or diarrhea, as dehydration increases the risk of kidney problems.

- Liver problems: Saxenda has not been extensively studied in individuals with liver problems. If you have a liver problem, it is advisable to consult your doctor to determine if Saxenda is appropriate for you.

- Depression or suicidal thoughts: In rare cases, individuals have reported experiencing suicidal thoughts or actions while taking Saxenda. If you have a history of depression or suicidal thoughts, or if you have experienced these issues in the past, it is important to discuss with your doctor whether Saxenda is suitable for you. It is also recommended to inform your doctor if you have had any other mental health conditions.

- Gastroparesis: Saxenda can cause gastroparesis, which is a condition characterized by slow stomach emptying. While Saxenda has not been studied in individuals with gastroparesis, it may potentially worsen the condition if you already have it. It is advisable to consult your doctor to determine if Saxenda is appropriate for you.

- Pregnancy: Saxenda is not safe to use during pregnancy. For more information, please refer to the "Saxenda and pregnancy" section above.

- Breastfeeding: It is unknown whether Saxenda is safe to use while breastfeeding. For more information, please refer to the "Saxenda and breastfeeding" section above.

Saxenda Expiration, Storage, and Disposal Guidelines

When you receive Saxenda from the pharmacy, the pharmacist will indicate an expiration date on the packaging label. Typically, this date is set to one year from the date of dispensing.

The expiration date is important as it ensures the medication's effectiveness within that timeframe. The Food and Drug Administration (FDA) advises against using expired medications. If you have any unused Saxenda that has exceeded the expiration date, consult your pharmacist for proper disposal instructions.

Storage

The duration of a medication's effectiveness can vary based on various factors, including storage conditions.

For new and unused Saxenda pens, it is recommended to store them in a refrigerator at a temperature between 36°F to 46°F (2°C to 8°C). It is crucial to prevent the pens from freezing, so do not use a pen that has been frozen.

Once you have started using a Saxenda pen, you can continue storing it in the refrigerator or keep it at room temperature between 59°F to 86°F (15°C to 30°C). Ensure that the pen is kept away from heat and light. After each injection, remove the needle and replace the pen cap. Do not store the pen with a needle attached.

Once in use, Saxenda remains effective for 30 days when stored as described above. If there is any medication left in the pen after 30 days of use, it should be disposed of.

Disposal

After using a needle, it is important to dispose of it in an FDA-approved sharps disposal container. This prevents accidental ingestion or harm to others, including children and pets. You can purchase a sharps container online or inquire with your doctor, pharmacist, or health insurance company for guidance on obtaining one.

This article offers helpful tips on medication disposal, and your pharmacist can also provide information on how to properly dispose of your medication.

What is the cost of Saxenda without insurance?

Losing weight can be difficult, and sometimes lifestyle changes alone are not enough to reach your weight loss goals. In these cases, your healthcare provider may recommend adding a prescription medication like Saxenda (liraglutide) to your weight loss plan.

Saxenda is an injectable medication that helps with weight loss by reducing appetite and increasing feelings of fullness. It comes in a pre-filled pen that can be used multiple times.

However, Saxenda can be quite expensive, costing thousands of dollars per year, making it unaffordable for many people. Additionally, even though Saxenda is FDA approved for weight loss, it may not be covered by health insurance plans. Fortunately, there are strategies to reduce out-of-pocket costs for Saxenda.

The manufacturer's list price for Saxenda is approximately $1,350 for a 30-day supply. However, if you are paying without insurance or discounts, the cost may be higher due to markups at pharmacies.

According to GoodRx data, the retail price of Saxenda ranges from $1,590 to $1,660 for a pack of 5 pre-filled pens. Each pen contains 18 mg (3 mL) of the medication.

The amount you pay out of pocket depends on various factors, including the pharmacy location, where you live, your health insurance coverage, and the dosage of Saxenda you are prescribed. Different pharmacies may charge different prices for Saxenda, and neighboring towns may have varying costs for the same medication.

Insurance coverage for Saxenda varies depending on the plan. While some commercial health insurance plans may cover the cost of Saxenda, there may be specific requirements that need to be met first. Employer-sponsored health insurance plans in the U.S. generally do not cover weight loss medications like Saxenda, although some employers may offer coverage. It is important to check with your health plan to understand your coverage details and requirements.

Medicare does not cover Saxenda or other medications for chronic weight management. However, Medicare Part B may cover behavioral therapy for obesity if certain criteria are met.

Some state Medicaid programs may cover Saxenda, but weight loss medications are often excluded from coverage. If your state Medicaid program covers Saxenda, there may be specific criteria and requirements to qualify for coverage.

To get your insurance to cover Saxenda, you can reach out to your medical team and discuss if Saxenda is a suitable option for you. It is important to check your insurance plan's formulary to see if Saxenda is included and if any prior authorization is required. If a prior authorization is needed, your prescriber can request it from your insurance company. If your prior authorization is denied, you can file an appeal and work with your prescriber to advocate for coverage.

There are also ways to save money on Saxenda. Using a GoodRx coupon can help you compare prices at different pharmacies and potentially save 21% off the retail price. Filling a 90-day supply instead of a 30-day supply can lower overall costs and reduce trips to the pharmacy. Using funds from your HSA or FSA can also help save money. Shopping around and asking for samples from your prescriber are additional strategies to consider.

While there are currently no manufacturer coupons or patient assistance programs for Saxenda, it is recommended to periodically check the manufacturer's website for any new offers that may become available.

www.ingramcontent.com/pod-product-compliance
Lightning Source LLC
Chambersburg PA
CBHW071951210526
45479CB00003B/893